Not Your Granny's Menopause

A Guide to Understanding "The Change"

Donna G. Ivery, MD

Copyright 2024 Swiner Publishing Company. All rights reserved.
ISBN: 9798883110701

Table of Contents

Foreword 7
Introduction 8
   Purpose 8
   How to Use the Book 11
The Basics 13
The Details 37
Questions 80
The Emotional Part 92
Conclusion 97
Reference Lists 100
   Types of hormonal preparations 100
   Side effect profile for estrogens 100
   Specific hormones 101
   Herbal options 102
   Nutraceutical options 105
   Non-pharmaceutical remedies 106
Resources 107
   9 Tips for a Successful Physician Visit 107
   Menstrual Cycle Calendar 110
   Menopause Symptom Tracker 114
About the Author 116
Join the Movement 119

FOREWORD

First, I dedicate this book to my great-grandmother, Emma Lee, and my great-great-grandmother, Martha, who each died due to childbirth complications, and my great-grandmother, Pearlie, who died at the age of 36 during the flu epidemic of the 1900s. None of them ever had the opportunity to write the menopause chapter of their lives.

Second, to every patient who has ever said to me, "I don't know what is happening with me," I thank you for trusting me with your care and allowing me to help you through your menopausal transition. This book could not have been written without you including me in your life experiences and I am humbled and enriched by that reality.

Introduction

Purpose

This is NOT intended to be a scholarly presentation on the science of menopause. The average woman is neither interested in nor worried about the science of it all. She just wants to stop worrying and feeling miserable and be reassured that everything will be okay. This book is not designed to convince you that menopause is a disease for which you need a cure (it is not). This book is not designed to convince you that menopause is a mystical moment that requires you to transcend your earthly limitations in order to conquer it.

My motivation for writing this book is simple: to help as many women as possible understand what menopause is all about.

Not a week went by in my OB/GYN private practice without a patient coming in with questions and concerns regarding menopause. Some patients were terrified at the prospect of going into menopause, some couldn't wait, some mourned the loss of their fertility for many different reasons, and others were indifferent. There were even a lucky few who didn't "know what all the fuss is about," because their periods just stopped one day and that was that! There were so many varied experiences with menopause, but the commonality was that patients didn't seem to know what to expect. They may have struggled to get their questions answered about what was happening in their bodies. They often feared the impact that natural, spontaneous menopause would have on their lives.

I would like this book to change that. I want you to be able to use this book as a guide to help you understand what menopause is all about. I also want it to help you understand the options available for help with menopausal symptoms.

I would break down patients seeking help into three categories. The biggest group of patients were the ones who wanted a better understanding of what was happening during menopause and what to expect. They were looking for knowledge and guidance about when to worry, reassurance that they were normal, and that this wouldn't last forever. Many of these women asked about menopause during their well woman visits. They hadn't experienced enough changes or concerns to justify making a separate appointment for intervention, but they wanted to make sure they were covering their bases.

The next largest group of patients were the ones having symptoms that were drastically impacting their lives. Hot flashes, sleep disturbances, and vaginal dryness or pain with intercourse led the way! It was so common to have patients come into the office with these complaints that the staff automatically understood to schedule a full 20-minute visit for them. Women are already running their lives at 120 mph and really have no tolerance for disruption. Menopausal changes come along and interrupt sleep and normal functioning and their lives quickly get derailed. I spent the time assessing the needs and desires for intervention with this group. Usually there was diagnostic testing and definitive intervention with a follow-up in three weeks to see if we were on the right track. We tweaked where she was during the follow up and most times had great results.

The last group of patients were sent in by their significant other. This was the most entertaining group. They didn't really think anything was wrong, but their intimate partners felt that they were catching hell. My delicate dance went something like this: I'd ask, "Why did your husband/significant other want you to see me?" I usually got a laugh or snicker with their response, "Because he wants to know why I don't want to have sex anymore." Ahhh, no libido. The patient is indifferent. After all, sex is not the only thing she doesn't want to be bothered with these days. Her husband feels like she doesn't love him anymore and the dog hides whenever she comes home from work. The children, well, they are teenagers, so they come with an asterisk. Explaining menopause, explaining what is happening with these symptoms, and validating that the patient does not require intervention (unless, of course, she wants it) are the tasks at hand for this group.

For each of these groups, there was this vague awareness that things would change with their cycles at some point around 50, but the details were never clear. The realities hit in a way they hadn't expected. I don't want you to experience menopause by accident. Let's get you prepped for this journey.

How to Use the Book

Your internet searches and AI questions will provide you with all of the words ever written about menopause in the last 100 years. Some of that information is accurate, some is actually inaccurate, and most is opinion. For far too many of you, asking your physician about menopause leaves you no better off than before your visit. Being ignored, belittled, rushed, dismissed, or just prescribed a routine set of pills is not the help you need or seek.

Spontaneous, natural menopause is a normal and natural developmental stage in a woman's life. If you were born with functioning ovaries and they have never been removed or destroyed and you live long enough, you will experience spontaneous, natural menopause. It is not a disease. It cannot be prevented, treated, or cured. Symptoms can become significant enough for you to need or want some type of intervention. This book will discuss various interventions. The information in this book is to explain this process, not diagnose your particular condition or advise on any specific treatment for you. Reading this book does not mean I am treating, curing, or diagnosing your situation or condition. If you are in need of intervention, please seek help from your physician or healthcare provider. This book is not to be used as medical advice. It is to be used as a guide.

This book is a combination of my experience, my expertise, and my opinions about menopause from the perspective of someone who has helped thousands of women over a 28-year clinical career as an OB/GYN physician. I have certainly helped over a thousand women with their menopausal experiences and got great feedback that my counseling and intervention were helpful and reassuring to them. They each had their own unique experience with menopause and decisions were made that fit their individual needs. In order for you to have the "best" experience, you need to know what's happening and what options are available. I want this book to be a foundational piece for you in making that happen. Use this book as a reference point and as a guide. You may not find yourself ready to embrace menopause, but by the end of this book, you will have a clearer understanding of spontaneous natural menopause.

THE BASICS

WHAT?

Menopause or "The Change" is the name commonly used to describe the physiologic transition period in women that defines the shift in reproductive hormone production from a cyclic, high-hormone level to a low, steady-state hormone level. This marks the end of a woman's natural fertility. Levels of the main hormone, estradiol, gradually decrease. Progesterone typically is no longer produced, but testosterone remains near its usual level. The official medical term for this transition period is **the menopause transition. Perimenopause** starts with the first cycle whose timing is off by more than seven days and continues until the final menstrual cycle. **Menopause** is the term that describes the final menstrual cycle. **Postmenopause** is the time after the final menstrual cycle. The first two years after the final menstrual cycle is considered early postmenopause and the next 4 years are considered late postmenopause. After your transition is finished, that time is called the rest of your life.

Menopause marks the end of the ability to release an egg from the ovaries for pregnancy. But in order to understand this, we actually need to start with an explanation of the menstrual cycle.

The menstrual cycle is a routine cycle of changing hormone levels that are designed to support the ability to produce high levels of reproductive hormones, develop a thick, vascular lining in the uterus, release an egg from the ovary, have it travel into the tube for fertilization, and have the fertilized embryo implant in the uterus and sustain itself until the placenta grows large enough to sustain the pregnancy on its own. The entire purpose of the cycle is for fertility and early pregnancy support. A cycle "begins" in the brain where a chemical signal, **Follicle-Stimulating Hormone (FSH)**, is secreted into the bloodstream to stimulate the ovaries to produce more estradiol. Rising levels of estradiol cause growth in several follicles inside the ovaries. These follicles produce increasing levels of estradiol as they grow until one of the follicles begins to grow substantially bigger and faster than the other ones. Eventually, the estradiol levels are high enough to trigger the brain to send a different chemical signal, **Luteinizing Hormone (LH)**, to release the egg from the large dominant follicle; that's called ovulation. The cells left behind in the dominant follicle then begin to produce progesterone. Once an egg has ovulated, it travels into and through the tube on its way to the uterus. Fertilization occurs during the egg's journey through the tube. The growing fertilized egg is now called an embryo and will enter the uterus. Once in the uterus, the embryo will implant and cells in the outer portion of the embryo will start to grow and begin secreting a hormone called Beta HCG (the pregnancy hormone). As long as Beta HCG hormone is circulating in the blood within seven days of ovulation, the progesterone secreting cells will continue to produce hormones. This progesterone production is critical in maintaining the early pregnancy until the placenta can grow and support the pregnancy on its own. Usually, the placenta takes over full hormone production for the pregnancy around 8-10 weeks.

If there is no Beta HCG in the bloodstream seven days after ovulation, the cells in the ovary that are producing progesterone will automatically start to die off and stop producing progesterone. Once progesterone levels begin to return to zero, the lining of the uterus is triggered to start to separate and shed. This shedding is what we know as menstrual bleeding. This is a regular, natural and predictable cycle each month. As the number of working follicles in the ovaries decrease to almost nothing, the ovaries' ability to produce hormones becomes impaired. The brain responds by increasing the signals to the ovaries to make more estradiol. As the last remaining follicles/eggs are used, the ovaries no longer have the ability to produce estradiol or progesterone. There are not enough hormones around to support growth and development of the uterine lining which leads to cessation of menstrual bleeding. As the cells throughout the body start to experience consistent low levels of estradiol, the changes in function that occur trigger the classic symptoms that women experience in menopause.

WHO?

Now that you understand *what* is happening in your body, let's look at *who* it is happening to. Spontaneous natural menopause occurs in women (46XX humans), born with functioning ovaries, who remain alive long enough to run out of eggs available to ovulate. This is a natural function of aging in women.

Transgender men (46 XX, assigned female at birth) who have

not had their ovaries removed will go through spontaneous natural menopause even if they are on testosterone therapy.

A hysterectomy (surgical removal of the uterus) does NOT cause menopause. If the ovaries are not removed surgically AND they continue to function normally, then menopause has not occurred.

A uterine ablation (surgical procedure to stop the uterine lining from bleeding) does NOT cause menopause. The loss of menstrual cycle bleeding is due to the surgery, not a problem with the ovaries.

Surgical menopause (removal of the ovaries prior to natural menopause) and chemical menopause (medications that prevent or block the ovaries from producing hormones) are considered medical conditions. They are not naturally-occuring experiences and are generally managed by a physician.

WHEN?

Spontaneous natural menopause occurs at age 51. That is traditionally considered to be the average age when an American woman will experience her final menstrual cycle. Additional studies provide conflicting evidence regarding the accuracy of this number across all ethnic groups. Eighty percent of women will complete menopause between the ages of 45 and 55. Another 8-10% of women will complete menopause between the ages of 40 and 45 (**early menopause**) and between the ages of 55 and 60 (**late-onset menopause**). Less than 1% of women complete menopause before age 40; they have undergone **premature menopause** (premature ovarian failure). Women finishing menopause after age 60 are considered to have experienced **late menopause**, which represents less than 1% of women.

The onset age of menopause is genetic—it is preprogrammed in your DNA. Your lifestyle and behavior, however, can have a significant influence on your actual age of menopause. Women who smoke more than 10 cigarettes a day will go through menopause almost 18 months earlier than their natural programming would dictate. Studies regarding smoking were conducted using cigarette usage. It is not clear how regular vaping nicotine or smoking/vaping cannabis or other herbs will affect the age of menopause.

Studies suggest that moderate consumption (no more than one drink per day) of white or red wine or liquor were mildly associated with the delay of the onset of menopause by six months to a year. Beer was not associated with changes in the onset age of menopause.

Being underweight (<18.5 BMI), is consistently associated with an earlier age of menopause. Overweight and obesity (between 29 and 35 BMI) are associated with later age of menopause.

Age at the time of your first menstrual cycle (menarche) is not related to age at menopause.

Decreased blood flow to the ovaries is a risk factor for earlier menopause. This can happen due to decreased physical activity and a sedentary lifestyle, tubal ligation, uterine surgery, uterine artery embolization, or cardiovascular disease.

Having one to three births is associated with later onset of menopause compared to having no births, but more than three births does not further delay menopause.

Giving birth after age 39 is associated with later menopause.

Women in the South have an earlier onset of menopause compared to other regions of the USA.

Hormonal contraceptive usage does not affect the age of menopause.

WHY?

Humans and four species of whales are the only creatures on Earth that live a significant amount of their lives after reproduction is over. It is not clear why this is the case, but researchers propose that the benefit of living so long past reproduction has provided an increased survival advantage to the species. It is suspected that humans thriving on the planet is partially due to the influence of grandmothers help with providing resources for the children of their offspring.

From a more modern outlook, if you achieve menopause, that means you survived!! Your mother didn't take you with her when she died in childbirth. YOU didn't die from infection or malnutrition as an infant. YOU didn't die from infection or trauma as a child or teen. YOU didn't die in childbirth or during pregnancy or postpartum. YOU didn't die from cervical cancer in your 40s. Here in the USA, we don't think about these things now, because they don't happen very much anymore; but as recently as 70 years ago, this was routine. Our grandmothers were the first generation of women in the USA to not live such traumatic and short lives. We are the first generation to not worry about making it to menopause. What a blessing!

I know many don't believe me, but you can check your own family history. The 1870-1920 census records in the USA document a lot of these stories. Trace all of your great-grandmothers during that time period to see how many siblings and mothers gradually disappeared from those census records. The bottom line is that many women didn't live long enough to experience menopause back in the day. I want us all to give a shout out to the amazing impact of practical technology and medicine on our lives. We should all appreciate access to public sanitation, clean water, antibiotics, vaccinations, pap smears, prenatal care, blood banking, attended births, and surgical intervention in the face of abnormal and complicated pregnancies and labor. Now, I'm not saying these things are all perfect and don't need adjustments. I am just acknowledging that these are some of the most significant factors that have led to the lifespan of American women doubling over the last 70 years. That should be embraced even as we aim to fix the problems and deficiencies incumbent with this reality.

HOW?

If you understand how the reproductive hormones affect your body, then you'll understand why symptoms can occur. Our reproductive hormones are made from cholesterol consumed in our diet. **Estradiol** is the main hormone responsible for reproductive function in women and it is predominantly produced in the ovaries. The adrenal gland can also participate in small amounts of production, especially after menopause. Estradiol is broken down by the liver and generally eliminated from the body through the colon.

Let's look at some additional facts about estradiol:
- Estradiol promotes growth of breast tissue and glands.
- Estradiol supports growth and maturation of ovarian follicles (eggs and their hormone producing cells).
- Estradiol promotes growth of the uterine lining.
- Estradiol increases blood flow to the muscles and fascia of estrogen-sensitive tissues in the vagina, bladder, and pelvis.
- Estradiol increases sensitivity to insulin and stabilizes subcutaneous fat, but also increases metabolism to reduce visceral fat.
- Estradiol moderates the immune system and suppresses inflammation.
- Estradiol directly impacts Vitamin D metabolism and its effects on bone, the immune system, and the endovascular system.
- Estradiol has profound effects on neurologic function and mood. Neurotransmitter release, receptor binding, blood flow, and inflammation are all sharply affected by estradiol exposure.
- Estradiol has a direct effect on the type and function of gut bacteria present in the colon.
- Estradiol interacts directly with the endocannabinoid system to affect mood, anxiety, sleep, and inflammation.

Progesterone is produced mainly in the ovaries, but the adrenal gland can participate in small amounts of production, especially after menopause. Progesterone is a profoundly powerful hormone, especially with regard to sleep, mood, smooth muscle function, breast development, and placental support.

Let's look at some additional facts about progesterone:

- Progesterone promotes the development of the uterine lining to support implantation.
- Progesterone relaxes smooth muscles, like the uterus and the gastrointestinal tract.
- Progesterone promotes relaxation and calmness.
- Progesterone helps stimulate effective deep breathing.
- Progesterone supports the placenta during pregnancy.
- Progesterone suppresses ovulation to prevent additional eggs from being released during pregnancy.
- Progesterone enhances getting to sleep and staying asleep.
- Progesterone helps stabilize and repair brain and myelin injury.
- Progesterone provides support to the adrenal gland during times of stress to produce more cortisol.

The last of the big three reproductive hormones for women is **Testosterone**. Testosterone is not typically associated with ovulation and reproduction, but it has a profound impact on sexual function and mood. Testosterone is produced by the ovary, adrenal glands, skin cells, and fat cells. Women produce testosterone at low levels compared to men and those levels decline somewhat into middle age, then remain steady. It exists in the blood in a bound and freely circulating form.

Let's look at some additional facts about testosterone:

- Testosterone contributes to a sense of well-being.
- Testosterone increases libido.
- Testosterone increases bone density.
- Testosterone increases oil production and lubrication.
- Testosterone increases hair growth and thickness.
- Testosterone increases muscle development and increases metabolism.
- Testosterone increases motivation and energy.
- Testosterone is converted into an estrogen (estrone) in adipose tissue.

These are the three primary reproductive hormones in women but not the only hormones of concern. The massive changes in your reproductive hormones during menopause will put stress on all of your other hormonal and regulatory systems: adrenal, thyroid, sleep, immune, and cardiovascular. In order to understand how menopause can disrupt your ENTIRE body, you must understand the importance of these other systems.

OTHER SYSTEMS

Adrenals

The adrenal glands are small, globs of fortune cookie shaped tissue sitting on top of each kidney. The adrenal glands have two different layers: the cortex and the medulla. The cortex produces three different sets of hormones, while the medulla produces adrenaline.

The outermost layer of the adrenal cortex primarily produces a hormone called aldosterone. Aldosterone is used by the kidneys to control blood pressure by balancing salt and water in the body. The middle layer primarily produces a hormone called cortisol. Cortisol mainly helps control how we respond to chronic stress in our lives, boosts our energy, influences how well your body responds to injury and inflammation, and contributes to maintaining our blood pressure. The inner layer primarily produces a hormone called Dehydroepiandrosterone (DHEA). DHEA is a precursor hormone in the ovaries and adrenal glands used for the production of other steroid hormones like estradiol, cortisol, progesterone, and testosterone.

The medulla produces adrenaline (epinephrine) to control your emergency "fight or flight" stress response. Adrenaline stimulates rapid changes like increasing the strength and speed of your heartbeat, dilating the pupils for sharper vision, opening your airways to increase the amount of oxygen that can get into your system, making you more alert and awake to enhance focus, and increasing blood flow to the arms, legs, and brain for enhanced functioning.

In summary, the adrenal gland system is responsible for producing hormones that are vital for our body's response to stress, regulating our blood pressure, managing our energy levels, and maintaining our overall balance. It helps us adapt to different situations and keeps our body and reproductive hormones functioning properly.

Thyroid

The thyroid gland is the small butterfly-shaped tissue located in the front of your neck. The thyroid gland's main job is to produce hormones that help regulate our body's metabolism. These two important hormones are Thyroxine (T4) and Triiodothyronine (T3). T4 and T3 hormones produced by the thyroid gland travel through the bloodstream to all areas of your body and influence almost every cell, tissue, and organ. They help regulate your heart rate, body temperature, and how you use energy. They also affect the growth and development of your body and brain, especially during childhood.

Sometimes, the thyroid gland can become overactive or underactive. When it's overactive, it produces too much hormone, leading to a condition called hyperthyroidism. This can cause symptoms like weight loss, rapid heartbeat, and feeling overly warm. On the other hand, when the thyroid gland is underactive, it doesn't produce enough hormone, leading to a condition called hypothyroidism. This can cause symptoms like fatigue, weight gain, and feeling cold.

Doctors can perform tests to measure the levels of T4, T3, and Thyroid-stimulating hormone (TSH) in the blood to determine if the thyroid gland is functioning properly. If any issues are found, there are treatments available to help restore the balance of thyroid hormones in the body.

In summary, the thyroid system plays a crucial role in regulating our body's metabolism, growth, and development. It produces hormones that affect many functions in our body, such as heart rate, body temperature, and energy use. When the thyroid gland isn't working correctly, it can lead to various symptoms, but with medical care, imbalances can be managed effectively.

Hypothalamus-Pituitary system

The pituitary gland sits at the base of the brain (behind the nose and between the eyes) directly connects to the hypothalamus via the pituitary stalk. The pituitary stalk consists of a network of nerves connected to the posterior pituitary lobe and blood vessels delivering hormones to the anterior lobe. Think of this interconnected system like a network dispatcher who assures that the glands are all functioning correctly and in sync. Specialized sensing neurons in the brain monitor hormone levels in the bloodstream and relay those levels to the hypothalamus. When there is a problem that needs correcting, the hypothalamus, which is the region of the brain that surrounds and stimulates the pituitary gland, "cranks up" or "calms down" the gland in question. The pituitary gland produces TSH, which tells the thyroid gland to make more or less T4 and T3 hormones based on the body's needs. The pituitary gland produces a hormone called adrenocorticotropic hormone (ACTH), which tells the adrenal gland to make more cortisol and DHEA. For the ovaries, the pituitary gland produces FSH to produce more estradiol and LH to induce ovulation. Prolactin is also secreted to increase milk production and growth hormone is secreted and affects growth and metabolism.

Other regions of the pituitary gland act to help rapidly adjust select systems and processes in the body. Oxytocin is released to support processes with labor (childbirth), breastfeeding (milk let-down), and sexual response (orgasm). Vasopressin, also known as antidiuretic hormone (ADH), is released in response to dehydration.

Sleep

There are several hormones that are involved in regulating our sleep-wake cycles and promoting healthy sleep. Two important hormones in this process are melatonin and cortisol.

Melatonin is often referred to as the sleep hormone, because it helps regulate our sleep-wake cycles. It is produced by a small gland in our brain called the pineal gland. Melatonin levels rise in the evening and remain high throughout the night, promoting feelings of sleepiness. This hormone is influenced by the amount of light we are exposed to. When it's dark, our body produces more melatonin, signaling that it's time to sleep. Exposure to bright light, especially blue light from electronic devices, can suppress melatonin production, making it harder to fall asleep.

Cortisol, often referred to as the stress hormone, also plays a role in our sleep-wake cycles and is produced by the adrenal glands. Cortisol levels naturally follow a daily pattern, with higher levels in the morning to help us wake up and lower levels in the evening to promote sleep. However, if we experience chronic stress or irregular sleep patterns, cortisol levels can become imbalanced and disrupt our sleep.

Other hormones that can impact sleep include **serotonin,** and **growth hormone.** Serotonin, known as the feel-good hormone, helps regulate mood and promotes feelings of relaxation and well-being. Adequate serotonin levels are important for healthy sleep. Growth hormone, produced by the pituitary gland, is involved in tissue repair and growth. It is primarily released during deep sleep, contributing to physical restoration and rejuvenation. Gamma-aminobutyric acid (**GABA)**, is a neurotransmitter, a substance that functions as a signal between nerve cells, that inhibits or buffers the response of other cells to neurotransmitters. Reducing the response to the neurotransmitters that stimulate and excite you are how it helps to regulate stress and sleep.

The hypothalamus plays a crucial role in temperature regulation. It acts as the body's thermostat, constantly monitoring the temperature and sending signals to make adjustments as needed. When our body temperature rises above the desired level, the hypothalamus triggers responses to cool down the body, such as increasing sweat production and dilating blood vessels near the skin's surface to release heat through water evaporation. Our symptoms of being hot are due to the way our body responds to reduce its internal temperature.

Conversely, when our body temperature drops below the desired level, the hypothalamus signals responses to warm up the body, such as shivering to generate heat and constricting blood vessels to reduce heat loss.

Thyroxine and adrenaline (epinephrine) are hormones that play a role in this process too. Thyroxine helps regulate our body's metabolism, including how quickly we burn energy and generate heat. When we encounter a stressful or threatening situation, adrenaline is released into our bloodstream. Adrenaline helps increase our heart rate, blood pressure, and breathing rate, but can also cause blood vessels in our skin to constrict, reducing blood flow to the skin's surface and helping to conserve heat. This stress response can temporarily increase our body temperature.

Mood and menopause

Mood refers to your emotional state or how you feel at any given time. Your mood can vary throughout the day, influenced by various factors. Your mood can vary over time, leading to changes, like depression and anxiety, that can significantly interfere with how you function. Mood is very complex and can be influenced by many factors, including gut health, hormone levels, neurotransmitter levels, life experiences, and external events.

Neurotransmitters are chemical messengers, manufactured in our gastrointestinal lining (gut) and in our brain, that help transmit signals between nerve cells. Two important neurotransmitters involved in regulating mood are serotonin and dopamine.

Serotonin is associated with a positive mood and a sense of calmness. Low levels of serotonin have been linked to feelings of sadness, anxiety, and even depression.

Dopamine is important in motivation, focus, and feelings of satisfaction.

GABA is associated with relaxation, calming, and reduction in feelings of fear, irritability, and anxiety.

Hormones also contribute to regulating mood. Estradiol has a profound effect on the secretion and availability of mood stabilizing neurotransmitters like serotonin and dopamine. This leads to feelings of happiness, warmth, desire to interact, and calmness. Progesterone also exhibits significant impact on mood through GABA influences to cause sedation and reduced anxiety. Testosterone enhances well-being, confidence, and sex drive. Chronically elevated cortisol levels can negatively impact mood and contribute to feelings of anxiety and irritability. Oxytocin is associated with feelings of love, empathy, and well-being. It can contribute to a positive mood and a sense of happiness.

Immune system changes

Estrogen plays a role in regulating the immune system. It helps enhance immune responses and has anti-inflammatory properties. One of the changes that may occur in the immune system during menopause is a decrease in the body's ability to fight off infections. Additionally, the decrease in estrogen levels can disrupt the balance in the distribution and function of immune cells.

Menopause can also be associated with an increased risk of worsening or new onset of certain autoimmune diseases. Menopause can impact the immune system, which is a complex network of cells and processes that is also influenced by other factors, such as overall health, genetics, and lifestyle.

Metabolism changes

Metabolism refers to the processes in our body that convert food into energy. One of the primary reasons metabolism can be affected during menopause is the decrease in estrogen. Estrogen helps maintain the balance between body fat and muscle mass, and it also influences how our body stores and uses energy (fat).

With the decline in estrogen levels during menopause, some women may experience changes in their body composition. They may notice an increase in body fat, particularly around the abdomen, and a decrease in muscle mass. This shift in body composition can lead to a decrease in basal metabolic rate (BMR), which is the amount of energy our body needs to perform basic functions at rest. A lower BMR means that the body requires fewer calories to maintain its basic functions, which can contribute to weight gain or make it harder to lose weight.

In addition to the reproductive hormone changes, other factors can also contribute to changes in metabolism during menopause. Aging itself can lead to a gradual decrease in metabolic rate through lower amounts of growth hormone and reduced secretion of thyroid hormone. Lifestyle factors, such as increased chronic stress, decreased physical activity, poor diet, accumulated exposure to toxins, and changes in sleep patterns may also influence metabolism during this stage of life.

It's important to note that while some women may experience significant changes in metabolism during menopause, not all women have this problem.

After menopause, in addition to the changes in estrogen levels, other factors can affect metabolism, including insulin resistance and thyroid hormone.

Insulin is a hormone produced by the pancreas that helps

regulate blood sugar levels. Insulin resistance occurs when the body's cells become less responsive to the effects of insulin. This means that the body needs to produce more insulin to help control blood sugar levels. Insulin resistance can lead to difficulties in maintaining normal blood sugar levels and can contribute to weight gain. After menopause, the decrease in estrogen levels can contribute to insulin resistance. This can lead to weight gain, particularly around the abdomen.

Another factor that can impact metabolism after menopause is the thyroid; hypothyroidism can occur more frequently during this stage. Hypothyroidism can lead to a decrease in metabolic rate, causing weight gain and feelings of fatigue.

On the other hand, some women may experience an autoimmune condition called Hashimoto's thyroiditis, which can cause inflammation and damage to the thyroid gland. This can also lead to changes in thyroid hormone levels. If a woman has concerns about insulin resistance, thyroid health, or experiences significant changes in weight or metabolism after menopause, it is advisable to consult with a physician or other healthcare professional who can provide personalized guidance, conduct appropriate tests, and recommend appropriate interventions.

Cardiovascular system changes

Estrogen plays a protective and anti-inflammatory role in the cardiovascular system by helping maintain healthy blood vessels and contributes to a favorable lipid profile (cholesterol and fats in the blood). Estrogen also has anti-inflammatory properties, which can help protect the blood vessels from damage and reduce the risk of cardiovascular diseases. The decline in estrogen after menopause can have very significant effects on the cardiovascular system. Some of the changes that can occur include:

1. Increased risk of cardiovascular disease. After menopause, the risk of developing cardiovascular diseases, such as heart disease and stroke, increases. Estradiol typically contributes to the relaxation and flexibility of blood vessels. Blood vessels are also more protected from damaging inflammation in the presence of estradiol.

2. Changes in lipid profile. Menopause can lead to increases in low-density lipoprotein (LDL) cholesterol, often referred to as "bad" cholesterol, and decreases in high-density lipoprotein (HDL) cholesterol, often referred to as "good" cholesterol. These changes can contribute to the buildup of fatty deposits in areas of inflammation in the blood vessels, increasing the risk of heart disease.

3. Changes in blood pressure and blood vessel function. The blood vessels may become less flexible and more prone to stiffness and inflammation after menopause. This can impair their ability to expand and contract efficiently, affecting blood flow and increasing the risk of cardiovascular problems.

Sleep

Sleep plays an important role in our overall health and well-being, including our weight. Getting enough good-quality sleep is essential for maintaining a healthy weight and supporting weight loss efforts. When we sleep, our bodies and brains undergo important processes that, likewise, help regulate our emotions and moods. Sleep allows our brains to rest, recharge, and process the events and experiences of the day. It helps restore the balance of chemicals in our brains that influence our mood and emotions. When we sleep, our bodies perform various important functions. The most critical of these tasks occurs during the periods of deep sleep. These include processing memory, adjusting caloric expenditure, regulating hormones that affect our appetite and metabolism, adjusting hormone secretion patterns, and removing waste from the brain. In addition to hormonal changes, insufficient sleep can also affect our energy levels and motivation to engage in physical activity.

Sleep also plays a role in managing stress. When we're well-rested, we're better equipped to cope with daily challenges and stressors. Adequate sleep supports our ability to think clearly, problem-solve, and make decisions, which can contribute to a more positive mood and better emotional well-being. Sleep and mood are intimately connected and dependent on each other. Poor sleep can contribute to negative moods, which can disrupt sleep. This can create a cycle where sleep problems and mood disturbances reinforce each other.

High blood pressure and menopause

Hypertension, or high blood pressure, is a condition in which the force of blood against the walls of the arteries is consistently too high. When estrogen levels decrease during menopause, it can lead to changes in the blood vessels. The blood vessels may become less flexible and more prone to stiffness, known as endothelial dysfunction. This stiffness causes resistance to blood flow and the blood pressure to rise.

Additionally, hormonal changes during menopause can contribute to weight gain and redistribution of body fat. The excess weight, especially around the abdomen, can increase the workload on the heart and blood vessels, raising blood pressure.

Stroke and menopause

The majority of strokes occur because there is existing damage and plaque formation (atherosclerosis) in the blood vessels of the brain. If a blood clot forms in one of the vessels supplying blood to the brain, it can deprive the brain cells of oxygen and nutrients, leading to a stroke. This loss of blood flow to a part of the brain leads to brain cell damage that can be permanent.

Estrogen helps keep blood vessels flexible and relaxed, promoting healthy blood flow to the brain and reducing the risk of blood clots. When estrogen levels decrease during menopause, it can lead to the blood vessels becoming less flexible and more prone to stiffness and damage. The increase in inflammation from this damage can increase the risk of blood clots forming within the vessels.

Additionally, other factors that commonly occur during menopause, such as elevated cholesterol (low density lipoproteins or triglycerides) levels, and the presence of other medical conditions, like uncontrolled high blood pressure (hypertension) or diabetes, can also contribute to the increased risk of stroke.

The Details

Being able to talk about menopause in a way that everyone understands is difficult. The most frustrating aspect of it is the limited ability to predict when a woman will permanently stop having menstrual cycles, menopausal symptoms, and pregnancies. The original attempts to standardize the way in which we communicate about menopause were published in the 1950s. There have been many studies attempting to characterize all aspects of the menopause transition. Infertility treatment and research highlighted the need for improvements in laboratory testing standards and consistency in communicating the stages of ovarian aging and function. The STRAW +10 protocol was formulated to answer this need. It is a standardized, objective set of terms that looks at changes in the timing of menstrual cycles (not changes in the amount of blood flow), blood testing of FSH, Anti-Mullerian hormone (AMH), and inhibin B, ultrasound assessment of antral follicle count, and presence of vasomotor symptoms (hot flashes) and/or genitourinary complaints. Age is not a component of this staging criteria. There are eight stages in this protocol. Understanding the details of each stage is not more important than understanding what we call different phases of the menopausal transition. **Premenopause** (stages -5, -4, and -3) is full ovarian function with no changes in menstrual frequency, no vasomotor symptoms, and reproductive levels of bloodwork and ultrasound findings. **Perimenopause** (stages -2, -1) starts with the first time the menstrual cycle occurs more than seven days early, more than seven days late, or skips a full 30 days in a female with regular and predictable cycles. There may be no vasomotor symptoms initially, but late perimenopause usually produces vasomotor symptoms and menstrual cycles that are consistently more than seven days different from the regular cycles OR cycles skipping 60 days or more. The late phase of perimenopause typically lasts one to three years. The perimenopause phase ends with the final menstrual cycle. The final menstrual cycle is considered **menopause** (stage 0). **Postmenopause** (stages +1, +2, +3) is the time after the final menstrual cycle. The early phase of postmenopause (stage +1) is the first two years after the final menstrual cycle when vasomotor symptoms are still common and hormone levels will be low but still fluctuate to some degree. The late phase of postmenopause (stage +2) occurs over the third to sixth year after the final menstrual cycle. It's characterized by stable, very low blood levels of hormone. Most symptoms of menopause are resolving but there are increasing complaints of genitourinary symptoms. Stage +3 is after completion of the sixth year since the final menstrual cycle. This is the rest of a woman's natural life.

Storytime

Hot flashes bothered me until they didn't. I will be the first to tell you that I am fortunate to have had the ability to control, well, actually dominate, all the thermostats in my life. My bout with hot flashes wasn't even about flashes. I was simply uncomfortably hot ALL THE TIME. Day in and Day out, I was really hot. I wasn't really sweating as much as I was just feeling uncomfortably hot. I wanted to strip off all of my clothes, just stand around in a cool shower, and constantly drink ice water—it was awful! I tried to get a remote starter for my car so that I could avoid the five minutes it took to cool the hot interior down. That failed because the car was a manual transmission and I thought about ditching the car. I then realized that if the air around me could stay cooler, I could function. I soon discovered that 72° was a great setting, so the thermostats at home and in the office were set to that temperature. In all fairness, my child and my staff were not happy. I bought individual ceramic heaters for each workstation and exam room in the office and authorized a jacket and sweater as part of the uniform in the office. My child wore his long flannel pajamas at night and had a blanket on his bed. This made them all comfortable, and I could function again!!

Being in a position to control the environment around you goes a long way towards managing symptoms in a practical manner. For instance, you may not be able to control the thermostat in your work setting, but perhaps you can have a cooling fan for your workstation. You can reduce triggers by reducing alcohol intake, excess sugar intake, and caffeine intake. You can improve your hydration status. Make it a point to drink 2 liters (66 ounces) of water every day.

Symptoms

More than 85% of women have some set of symptoms to accompany their transition to menopause. The earliest changes happen with increasing PMS symptoms like mood disturbances and migraine headaches. The cycle may also change in frequency, duration, and amount. Women approaching menopause have higher rates of early pregnancy loss (before 10 weeks) and late term loss (after 36 weeks). The most common symptoms are hot flashes and/or night sweats, changes in menstrual bleeding pattern, sleep disturbance, mood changes, vaginal dryness, and decreased libido. Please do not look at this list as comprehensive; there are a MILLION other symptoms that can be associated with normal menopause. This simply covers the most common and familiar ones.

- Vasomotor symptoms:
  - <u>The Scenario:</u> **Hot flashes** are the sudden and unpredictable feeling of being **REALLY HOT**. Like burning up hot. Like "living in an oven" hot. Like being **"afraid you may burst into flames"** hot. It is often accompanied by sweating and water pouring down your forehead, your back, your armpits, and your thighs. Anywhere sweat forms, it pours. When this happens at night, it is called **night sweats**. When it is accompanied by turning red (in lighter skin complexions), it is called **flushing**. It

may be accompanied by nausea, palpitations, lightheadedness, and difficulty concentrating. You can feel dizzy, faint, or off balance. There are times when these hot flashes are then followed by chills. Hot flashes can last seconds to hours. You may **feel hot** all of the time. All of these things fall under the category of vasomotor symptoms.

- <u>Why it happens:</u> The area in the brain that controls internal body temperature is located in the hypothalamus next to the area that controls the ovaries. One of the chemical signals released from this area of the hypothalamus is **neurokinin B (NKB)**. The hypothalamus upregulates its functioning when hormone levels fall during the menopause transition. Increased secretion of NKB can also make the temperature control centers in the brain more unstable. Very mild stimulation can trigger the start of a cooling cycle in the body even though the internal temperature is normal. Blood vessels in the skin dilate to release heat and sweat glands open to release moisture that then evaporates from the skin to cool it down. The heart beats faster to deliver more blood to the skin for cooling. This feels the same as you would feel if your body temperature was actually elevated. 80% of women experience vasomotor symptoms. Symptoms may last from 5-12 years. There are a small number of women who have persistent symptoms throughout the remainder of their lives.

- Options:
  - You can take measures to make the environment cooler, like handheld and misting fans, cooling cloths, cooling pads, ice packs, cold drinks, and lowering the air temperature
  - Avoidance of triggers like alcohol and caffeine, other stimulants, increased stress, spicy foods, and hot environments
  - Hormonal therapy: estrogens and progesterone
  - Prescription therapy (approved): fezolinetant, and conjugated estrogens/bazedoxifene
  - Prescription therapy (off-label usage): gabapentin, SSRIs, SNRIs, and oxybutynin
  - Mind-body techniques: meditation, yoga, tai chi, and qi gong
  - Acupuncture/Acupressure
  - Procedure: Stellate ganglion block
  - Herbal or nutritional: soy isoflavones, ginseng, black cohosh/dong quai, evening primrose, red clover, rhapontic rhubarb, pine bark, red raspberry, and Vitex (chasteberry)

- Pain/Discomfort during intercourse:
  - The Scenario: **"It feels like sandpaper when I have sex."** That was the absolute most common vaginal

complaint I fielded in my OB/GYN practice when it came to menopause. Other descriptions were, "**My vagina feels dry**" or "**It hurts to have sex.**" Typically, some husbands said, "**It feels like I'm hitting a wall,**" "**I can tell it is hurting her,**" or "**It's not sliding like it usually does.**" All of these complaints fall under the category of genitourinary syndrome.

- <u>Why it happens:</u> The lining of the vagina is a type of skin tissue called epithelium, which is designed to be moist and stretchy. High estradiol levels cause increased blood flow to the lining of the vagina to support elasticity (stretchiness) and secretions for moisture, lubrication, and protection from injury. As estradiol levels fall during the transition to menopause, reduced blood flow leads to decreasing secretions. The first indication of this is the feeling of dryness or scratchiness during intercourse. As low estradiol levels continue over time, the reduced blood flow leads to a thinning of the vaginal lining and a loss of elasticity. When the vagina loses its "stretchability", penetration is impaired, and this causes pain and discomfort. These changes can even lead to tears and bleeding in the vagina. These changes are persistent without intervention but can be reversed in most women with proper treatment.
- <u>Options:</u>
    - Increased use of lubrication (food-grade oil or silicone based)

- Increased time for arousal
- Avoidance
- Vaginal moisturizers
- Hormonal therapy: estrogens, DHEA, and testosterone
- Prescription therapy (approved): Ospemifene
- Pelvic floor physical therapy
- Intermittent vaginal dilation
- Laser resurfacing or rejuvenation
- Plasma-rich platelet injections
- Herbal or nutritional: soy isoflavones, ginseng, black cohosh, evening primrose, red clover, rhapontic rhubarb, pine bark, red raspberry, and Vitex (chasteberry)

- **Changes in menstrual cycles:**
  - <u>The Scenario:</u> Patients would say, "**My cycle is heavier,**" "**I missed my last four periods,**" "**I skipped my last two months and now my cycle's been on for three weeks,**" "**My period keeps coming too soon,**" "**My bleeding is lasting longer,**" or "**My flow is shorter than it used to be.**" All of these complaints are common during the transition to menopause. These fall under several different terms like

menorrhagia, hypermenorrhea, hypomenorrhea, or irregular menses.

- <u>Why it happens:</u> As the ovaries begin to lose the ability to produce high levels of estradiol, the brain intensifies the signals to boost production. It is quite common for there to be fluctuating surges in hormones from cycle to cycle. Fluctuating hormone levels can then trigger changes in the timing of a menstrual cycle. If estradiol levels are somewhat low, it may take longer for an egg to mature enough to ovulate. This can lead to a longer or missed cycle. If estradiol levels are suddenly higher than normal, the cycle can trigger ovulation early. If progesterone levels are lower, this can limit how thick the uterine lining gets. It is also very common for women, especially in the USA, to have non-cancerous tumors in the uterus called fibroids. Fibroids are not caused by menopause, but symptoms can worsen during this time. Fluctuating levels of hormones can trigger changes in fibroids like rapid growth or degeneration. When going through the menopause transition, it is very common for women to present with heavier bleeding, increased pain, cramping, and anemia during their menstrual cycles. This often leads to a hysterectomy, the most common surgical procedure in women in the USA. Heavier or lighter bleeding, more frequent cycles, and skipped or delayed cycles are generally related to changes in hormonal levels associated with the menopause transition. Unpredictable bleeding, random spotting, and bleeding episodes that occur closer together than twenty-one days are all bleeding patterns that should be evaluated by your physician.

- Options:
  - Watch and wait
  - Cyclic combination hormone therapy (estradiol containing birth control pills)
  - Tranexamic acid (heavy bleeding)
  - Endometrial ablation (heavy bleeding)
  - Hormonal therapy: long-acting progesterone therapy (IUD, subdermal implant, and intramuscular injection)
  - Herbal or nutritional: soy isoflavones, red clover, red raspberry, and Vitex (chasteberry)

- **Decreased libido**
  - <u>The Scenario:</u> The number one complaint of women's partners is the lessening or absence of sex and feelings of being unwanted and undesired. Women often then may harbor guilt and feel like something is wrong. Women also came in with complaints on their own about not feeling the urges to have sex as much as they used to have them.

Libido is your sex drive; that spontaneous desire to have sex. I've heard it referred to as that "tickle in your twat." This loss of libido is not the same as not enjoying sex. Anytime a woman came to me with this complaint, I would ask her, "When your partner can find you and get you excited, do you enjoy it?" Invariably (for those who thought it was good before menopause), they would laugh and say, "Yes." Many of them admitted to hiding from their partners when they got home from work, faking being asleep before their partner went to bed, or getting out of bed and getting dressed in the morning before their partner woke up, so they wouldn't have to deal with the issue of sex. They were clear that it wasn't that sex was bad or different, they just didn't care if they had it or not. They didn't want to be bothered, which was very different than it used to be.

o **Why it happens:** The ovaries, in general, produce the same amount of testosterone throughout your adult life. The amount of estradiol in your system is what affects the impact of that testosterone. Decreasing estradiol levels compared to your usual testosterone levels are more to blame. Many women find that their libidos stabilize and improve after they achieve menopause and hormone levels stabilize. When their body gets accustomed to low estradiol levels, the testosterone effects start to kick back in.

- **Options:**
  - Schedule intercourse
  - Hormonal therapy: estrogen and testosterone combinations
  - Herbal or nutritional: horny goat weed, ginseng, fenugreek, maca, tribulus, or coffee
  - Increase sleep
  - Evaluate contraceptive choice if progesterone, only
  - Evaluate side effect from other medications like SSRI, SNRI, sedatives

Brain Fog

- **The Scenario:** Patients would say, **"I can't concentrate," "My brain is not working right," "I think I have Alzheimer's," "I got diagnosed with ADD!!" "I can't remember things," or "I can't get my work done."** Feeling like you are losing brain function is one of the scariest symptoms. Many women, especially women who have critical responsibilities in their lives, are distressed and panicky in the face of a brain that isn't working like it used to work. Brain fog incorporates symptoms like poor focus, slower mental processing, being easily distracted, difficulty with recall, difficulty learning new material, and difficulty organizing tasks.

o <u>Why it happens:</u> The role of estradiol and progesterone in the brain contributes to so many aspects of healthy function in women. During the transition to menopause, the loss of these hormones affects brain function in multiple ways. Insulin resistance decreases glucose (sugar) usage by brain cells, inflammation increases, blood flow decreases, and direct stimulation of nerve function decreases. Interrupted sleep patterns interfere with mood and memory. Disrupted hydration and electrolyte balance due to increased sweating directly affect brain cell function. The issue of brain fog is also a reminder that other things are going on in your life besides menopause. At midlife, approximately age 45-50, there are several other physiologic and lifestyle realities to address. Growth hormone is decreasing, the secretion of melatonin and cortisol are declining, home life may be transitioning from marriage to divorce, or child rearing to empty nesting. Financial concerns may come into play as the awareness or arrival of retirement, stagnant wage growth, divorce, death, college costs, and supporting adult children may occur. Parents may now need assistance and caregiving support. Health concerns due to lack of physical activity, obesity, high blood pressure, poor nutrition, and diabetes commonly present at this time, playing an active role in challenging brain function.

- Options:
  - Improve sleep
  - Maintain good hydration
  - Hormonal therapy: estrogens, DHEA, testosterone, or pregnenolone
  - Use digital or personal assistants for scheduling, reminders, and organization
  - Increase exposure to early morning sunlight or use a light box
  - Herbal or nutritional: gingko, ginseng, caffeine, lion's mane mushroom, MACA, green tea/EGCG, omega III, or CoQ-10

Storytime

I had taken a "new" patient for outpatient laparoscopic surgery (which was successful), but her husband wasn't present. It is very unusual in my experience for a married patient to have surgery and her husband not be available in the waiting room when I am finished. In this instance, the patient's Mother-in-law was present but all information was to be communicated to the husband. I called him to let him know the results of the surgery and he was very flippant in his response. He was actually a bit irritated that I had disturbed him during his working hours. The next thing you know, I hear this voice that sounds just like mine, telling him that he is being derelict in his duty as a husband to be present for his wife. He audibly gasped. He asked me what kind of doctor I was. I shot back that the question is what kind of husband is he that he didn't bother to come be with his wife during her surgery! Now, my unfiltered self was clearly in full control during this exchange while my mature and professional inner self was clear that I was out of control. I kept telling myself to pull back. That this wasn't me, that there was nothing good that could come from this behavior. He and I went back and forth a little while longer, but I eventually started tempering my behavior and successfully defused the situation. Once I calmed down and thought about what happened (hours later), I was mortified. I couldn't believe that I had done that. It was not as though that was the first time a husband had ever been a bonehead. But it was the first time that I had reacted to one like he was a bonehead and I didn't care if he knew it. THERE IS NOTHING GOOD THAT COMES OUT OF THAT BEHAVIOR. After this incident, I decided to try hormone therapy.

Some symptoms of menopause may be significant and not be bothersome enough to you for you to seek intervention. Other symptoms of menopause may be actively distressing and detrimental in your life. Recognizing when you need to get help is very important. You get no points for suffering and you may find yourself regretting your actions.

- Unpredictable mood changes: edginess, depression, and/or anxiety
    - <u>The Scenario:</u> So many women during the transition to menopause describe being "unable to control or predict how they feel or react." This often leads to loss of confidence in their ability to function, embarrassment, feeling like they are losing their minds, feeling like they are going crazy, and feeling like they are losing themselves. These feelings present in several different ways: increased anxiety and worry over insignificant things, debilitating anxiety and worry over big things in life like problems in a marriage or difficulty managing children and their behavior. Women indicated that they experienced uncontrollable crying, inappropriate anger, social withdrawal because they just can't stand to be around other people, declining assignments or travel at work because of the inability to trust themselves to be able to get the job done, or inappropriate communications and interactions with co-workers.

    - <u>Why it happens:</u> Multifactorial mechanisms again come into play regarding mood instability. Falling estradiol levels and absent progesterone levels each exert a direct effect on the centers of the brain that control emotions. Interruptions in sleep patterns are the next biggest contributor to mood changes. The worsening of pre-existing challenges with depression, anxiety, or other mental illness play a notable role in the manifestation of mood changes for many women during the transition to menopause.

- Options:
  - Regular sleep schedule
  - Increase exposure to early morning sunlight
  - Use a light box to mimic sunlight exposure
  - Stress reduction
  - Hormonal therapy: estrogens and progesterone
  - Prescription therapy (approved): SSRI, SNRI, and benzodiazepine
  - Cranial electrical stimulation
  - Meditation
  - Journaling
  - Counseling
  - Aromatherapy with essential oils: lavender, vanilla, jasmine, ylang ylang, lemongrass, bergamot, or frankincense
  - Herbal or nutritional: chamomile, lemon balm, L-theanine, CBD (edible)

- Sleep changes

    - <u>The Scenario:</u> You go to bed with the fan on high and AC cranked up. You still wake up feeling hot and kick the covers off. Then you wake up feeling cold and wet from sweating and take off your wet nightgown and put the covers back on. You wake up feeling hot again and kick the covers back onto the floor. This vicious cycle continues a few more times before 5 am. You finally get back to a comfortable sleep, but the alarm goes off at 6 am. It's easy to understand what is happening here; hot flashes and night sweats are disturbing your sleep. Another scenario is to be wide awake, every night between 2:30 and 3:30 am, like clockwork. You are awake and alert as if it is morning. This happens, predictably, every night. What is happening here is more related to anxiety and stress. The scenario that you probably never hear about is when you can't get to sleep or have a good deep sleep. You lay down feeling sleepy but can't fall asleep. You fall asleep but wake up from any little noise or movement. You "sleep" all night, but don't feel refreshed, because you never had a deep sleep. Not many women know that this is a very common scenario during menopause transition.

    - <u>Why it happens:</u> Hot flashes and night sweats that interrupt sleep tend to occur due to decreased estradiol levels. Awakening in the middle of the night at a predictable time is generally associated with abnormal cortisol secretion when the circadian rhythm is thrown off by chronic and significant stress. Difficulty falling asleep or falling into a deep sleep is directly related to the loss of the sedative and calming effect of progesterone. During the menopause transition, progesterone levels fall to almost zero and many women struggle with getting to sleep.

- Options:
  - Regular sleep schedule
  - Stop eating and drinking 2-3 hours before bed
  - Decrease noise and lights two hours before bed
  - Use your bedroom for sleep, dressing, and intimacy only—move all other activities to a different room
  - Address your sleep apnea/snoring
  - Address partner's sleep apnea/snoring
  - Stress reduction
  - Hormonal therapy: progesterone
  - Prescription therapy (approved): benzodiazepines (like valium, xanax, or ativan), barbiturates (seconal or nembutal), GABA agonists (like ambien, lunesta, or sonata), melatonin-receptor agonists

- Prescription therapy (off-label usage): amitriptyline or gabapentin
- Cranial electrical stimulation
- Meditation
- Journaling
- Sleep-inducing devices
- Counseling
- Over-the-counter: antihistamines
- Aromatherapy with essential oils lavender, vanilla, jasmine, ylang ylang, lemongrass, bergamot, or frankincense
- Herbal or nutritional: chamomile, lemon balm, melatonin, L-theanine, or cannabinol (oral)

- **Weight gain**
  - <u>The Scenario:</u> Oh, the dreaded menopause belly!!! Piling on weight in the midst of struggling with hormone levels sounds like torture. In addition to gaining weight, the distribution of weight shifts more towards the abdomen during the menopause transition. Maintaining lean muscle mass may also be compromised and previously successful weight loss methods may now fail. Weight gain during the menopause transition is not inevitable or uncontrollable, but it is very, very common.
  - <u>Why it happens:</u> Weight gain during

menopause can be attributed to many factors. Decreasing estrogen levels can increase insulin resistance. Midlife changes that impact growth hormone and thyroid hormone secretion can reset the basal metabolic rate and cause you to burn fewer calories. Sleep disruption has a very negative effect on appetite and focus, leading you to be much less consistent with managing weight. Attempts to self-medicate, regarding sleep and anxiety, can lead to increased alcohol consumption, which increases calories. Issues of fatigue and stress can lead to sharply reduced physical activity, which then leads to weight gain.

- Options:
  - A regular sleep schedule
  - Stress reduction
  - Intermittent fasting
  - Intentional eating regimen: DASH, Mediterranean diet, or low glycemic load
  - Increase muscle-building physical activity
  - Prescription therapy (approved): semaglutide, orlistat, phentermine/topiramate, or naltrexone/bupropion
  - Group support programs
  - Review existing prescriptions for side effects
  - Food journaling

- Bariatric surgery
- Localized fat removal (liposuction or lipolysis)

- Migraine headaches
  - <u>The Scenario:</u> Headaches are a common sign that your menstrual cycle is about to start—that pressure deep in your head that then becomes a dull ache on one side, just behind the eye. Migraine headaches can be very debilitating. It is not unusual for some women to start getting headaches a day or two before their bleeding starts. This can be easily addressed once it is recognized.

  - <u>Why it happens:</u> The last day or two before menstrual bleeding begins is the point in the normal menstrual cycle where both estradiol and progesterone are at their lowest, at the same time. As the ovaries struggle to produce normal amounts of hormone, the amount of hormone at the end of the cycle decreases as well. Low levels of estradiol are associated with increased tightening (constriction) of blood vessels, which can be associated with increased headaches.

  - <u>Options:</u>
    - A regular sleep schedule
    - A regular eating schedule

- Maintain good hydration
- Stress reduction
- Avoidance of triggers
- Acupuncture or acupressure
- Over-the-counter medications: aspirin, ibuprofen, or acetaminophen
- Prescription therapy (approved): Triptans (like Imitrex, Maxalt, or Zomig), ergotamines (like Fioricet), gepants (like Ubrelvy), monoclonal antibodies (like Aimovig or Emgality)
- Prescription therapy (off-label usage): estrogens, luteal-phase NSAIDS, or continuous combined hormonal therapy
- Relaxation techniques like yoga, biofeedback, or qi gong
- Hot or cold compresses for the head
- Massage
- Aromatherapy: lavender, peppermint, ginger, or rosemary
- Foods: AVOID foods high in nitrites, nitrates, tyramine, and gluten:

- **Osteoporosis**
  - <u>The Scenario:</u> Those visions of an elderly grandmother with a hunchback, unable to straighten up, are so

scary for many of us. The more common reality is an elderly parent or grandparent who is trucking along living their best life until a hip fractures and changes everything. Even now, 50% of elderly people who fracture a hip die within 6 months of the fracture, whether they get treated, have surgery, or not!

o <u>Why it happens:</u> Osteoporosis literally means porous (holey) bones. It is a normally occurring feature of aging. The speed and the amount of bone loss depends on many factors. Bones have three main functions:

- 1) Provide a rigid structure to support and protect the soft tissues of the body and allow movement.
- 2) A storage compartment for tissue that generates the cells in our blood (bone marrow).
- 3) An active storage form for the calcium required in the body. This calcium balance is critical for nerve signaling, muscle movement, blood clotting, cell secretion, and heart rhythm.

Bones are constantly under renovation with some cells building bone (osteoblasts) and some cells breaking bone down (osteoclasts). For females, one of the most critical factors is menopause. High estradiol levels trigger activity that favors the building of bone over the breakdown of bone. When estradiol levels remain low in menopause, the breakdown of bone becomes dominant and there is rapid bone loss. Females establish maximum bone density by age 30 and can lose 10-20% of their total bone density in the first 5 years after the final menstrual cycle. Osteopenia occurs when bone density is low enough to increase the risk of fracture under normal stressors and trauma. Osteoporosis occurs when bone density is so low that normal activity could lead to a fracture.

- Options:
  - Increase weight-bearing exercise
  - Increase muscle-building physical activity
  - Decrease stress
  - Stop smoking
  - Reduce alcohol consumption
  - Improve sleep
  - Tai chi
  - Acupuncture/Acupressure
  - Prescription therapy (off-label usage): testosterone supplementation, or combined estrogen and progesterone
  - Prescription therapy (approved): bisphosphonates, denosumab, estrogens, SERMs, calcitonin, romosozumab, abaloparatide, or teriparatide

- Food: decrease caffeine intake, eliminate cola intake, avoid consuming calcium at the same time as phytates (in beans and wheat bran), oxalates (in beets and rhubarb), and iron (in spinach)
- Herbal or nutraceutical: calcium, magnesium, vitamin D3, glucosamine chondroitin, vitamin K2, vitamin C, copper, zinc, strontium, manganese, silicon, or boron

- **Apathy**
  - <u>The Scenario:</u> Fatigue is a very common complaint during menopause. When patients had this complaint, the underlying problem was not always so clear. It is very easy to attribute fatigue to the dehydration and interrupted sleep that occur in a woman with significant sweating and hot flashes. Heavy or prolonged bleeding can lead to anemia which contributes to fatigue. Apathy and lack of motivation are very frequently assumed to be fatigue and are often missed (or ignored) symptoms of menopause. Patients would say, "I just don't want to do anything," "My laundry is piling up and my house is a mess and that's not like me," "I have all of these things to do at work but I can't make myself get them done," or "I am stressed because I am struggling to get up in the morning and get things done during the day!"

- <u>Why it happens:</u> Estradiol affects the areas in our brain that control dopamine balance. As estradiol levels get lower during menopause, dopamine levels can also drop. Low dopamine levels are associated with apathy (lack of goal-directed activity, lack of interest, and/or lack of emotional expression). Loss of libido is very likely a result of the apathy that can occur during menopause as opposed to being an isolated sexual dysfunction.

- <u>Options:</u>
  - Schedule activities and deadlines
  - Decrease stress
  - Improve sleep
  - Review prescriptions for side effects: SSRIs, anti-seizure meds, or anti-psychotic meds
  - Prescription therapy (off-label usage): testosterone supplementation, combined estrogen and testosterone, selegiline, amantadine, or aripiprazole
  - Foods: Dark chocolate, pumpkin seeds, avocado, watermelon, eggs, green tea, banana, green leafy vegetables, chicken, dairy, or fish

Storytime

I was asked to see a patient because she had missed her cycle. She was 53 years old and just didn't feel well. Her cycles had been regular up until several months ago and she hadn't had any since then. Her tubes had been tied for 30 years, so that wasn't the issue. She just didn't think she would feel so tired during menopause and wanted to make sure nothing was wrong. We ordered the standard lab blood tests for her and sure enough, her pregnancy test was positive. Very positive! Even though the results were reliable, we also waited for the actual quantitative hormone levels, and they were unequivocally positive. She was pregnant. I knew all of this before I met with her, because I hadn't been the first doctor she had seen that day. She simply wouldn't acknowledge what the first doctor had told her. I introduced myself and asked her why she had come to the office that day. She gave me the same history I had been told. I asked about her last menstrual period and she confirmed that it had been several months ago. I told her that her blood pregnancy test results were back and that she was in fact pregnant. She looked at me, blinked, turned her head, and then continued talking about how tired she was. I said, "Ma'am, you are not going through 'The Change', you are pregnant." Again, she looked at me, blinked, turned her head away from me, and continued talking about how she didn't think that being this tired happened during "The Change." I realized we had a problem, so I stopped her and asked her if she had **heard** me. She said, "Yes, I heard you, but you said I'm pregnant and that isn't possible because my tubes have BEEN tied!" I told her that I know she doesn't want to hear me, but that I had already verified that her urine and blood test results were positive. She let out a scream that would wake the dead. "NNNNNNOOOOOOOOOO!!!!" she shouted. I took a deep breath to gather my wits and reassured her that it was going to be alright. "IT'S NOT GOING TO BE ALRIIIGGGGHHTTTT!!!" she screamed. She collapsed onto the floor continuing to scream. I tried to encourage her to get up, but she kept rolling and wailing. I tried to calm her down and told to take a deep breath, but she started banging her head on the floor!! I got down on the floor with her and shouted into her ear, "That Is ENOUGH carrying on!! If you bang your head on the floor again, I will have the psych people come get you!!!" She, thankfully, stopped banging her head on the floor and looked me straight in my face and asked me, through her sobbing and crying, why I couldn't just tell her she had cancer? Whew, chile! I was speechless. I told her to let me help her get up off the floor and we'd figure out what to do. She got up still wailing and sobbing and sat down. It turned out that her granddaughter was also pregnant and there was simply no way she could fathom being pregnant after all of these years. She finally calmed down enough to function and listen. We got her set up for an ultrasound appointment immediately (she had a normal intrauterine pregnancy), had someone from her family come and pick her up, and made another appointment in a few days to address her options. From that day forward, I was always super aggressive with my patients over 45 about effective contraception during menopause. Given the repeal of Roe vs. Wade, this type of scenario is no longer a simple routine issue.

Please do not assume that you cannot get pregnant during the menopause transition. While your odds of getting pregnant get lower and lower as you get closer to your final menstrual cycle, there are never any guarantees.

- **Pregnancy**
  - **Description**: YES! You can get pregnant during the transition to menopause!! If you ovulate and have unprotected intercourse, you can get pregnant. If you don't know if you are ovulating and you have unprotected sex, you can get pregnant. 78% of pregnancies that occur in women over 40 are unintended.

  - **Why it happens:** Ovulation is unpredictable during the transition to menopause, but it can happen. Reduced fertility begins up to 10 years before the final menstrual cycle. As hormone levels get progressively lower, changes in bleeding during the menstrual cycle start to occur. It is possible to ovulate without bleeding the previous month when a female is in the menopause transition. Do not take chances, especially now that abortion is unavailable in so many states. Do NOT assume you can't get pregnant just because you haven't had a menstrual cycle in three or four months. FSH levels above 50 at the same time as LH levels above 40 in a woman who has gone a full 12 months without a cycle are consistent with having achieved menopause. In my practice, I would repeat these labs after an additional year before I felt comfortable telling a patient she could stop contraceptives or remove IUDs or Nexplanons. Review your specific situation with your gynecologist before making the decision to stop contraceptive practices.

- Options:
  - Abstinence
  - Partner sterilization
  - Sterilization
  - Intrauterine device
  - Subdermal implant
  - Birth control pills
  - Barrier contraception (condoms, spermicides)
  - Intravaginal hormonal ring

- ## Worsened PMS

  - <u>Description:</u> That time period that used to be three days before your cycle starts is now happening five days before your cycle starts. More cramping, more bloating, more grogginess, more irritability, and more moodiness. The earliest signs of hormonal fluctuations in the early stages of the transition to menopause occur in the premenstrual (luteal) phase of the cycle.

  - <u>Why it happens:</u> When the ability of the corpus luteum (progesterone secreting cyst left in the ovary after ovulation) to generate adequate progesterone gets compromised, the premenstrual symptoms can become more intense and occur earlier than they usually do in your cycle. More severe mood changes, increased sleepiness, and worsened bloating are all features affected by this earliest of hormonal changes.

- o Options:
  - ■ Prescription (approved): paroxetine, fluoxetine, or sertraline
  - ■ Prescription (off-label usage): birth control pills, IUD, etonogestrel implants, medroxyprogesterone acetate injections, or diuretics
  - ■ Light therapy
  - ■ Herbal or nutraceutical: magnesium, B6, peony, ginger, dandelion, fennel, black cohosh, dong quai, red raspberry leaf, saffron, St. John's Wort, or evening primrose

- **Dry eyes, dry mouth, and dry skin**
  - o The Scenario: Just like the vagina, the surface of the eyes and the lining of the mouth are types of skin tissue. Problems with chronically dry eyes, a dry mouth, and dry skin are quite common during the menopause transition. These concerns can become quite worrisome and lead to a need for intervention in many women.
  - o
  - o Why it happens: Decreased estradiol levels

lead to decreased blood flow to these layers of epithelium. Decreased blood flow leads to decreased secretions and thinning of the tissue, which lead to delicate tissues that are easily damaged and irritated.

- o <u>Options:</u>
  - Moisturizers
  - Eyes: lacrimal duct plugs
  - Topical oils to condition skin
  - Tri-peptide collagen
  - Hormonal therapy: estrogens, DHEA, testosterone
  - Herbal or nutritional: soy isoflavones, ginseng, black cohosh, evening primrose, red clover, rhapontic rhubarb, pine bark, red raspberry, Vitex, hyaluronic acid, or biotin

- Urinary leakage (incontinence)
  - o <u>The Scenario:</u> You have a little cough, a little laugh, or a little jump and now there is a little leak. Perhaps you already had a little urinary leakage, every now and then, but since you started your transition to menopause, it's happening a lot more. This is very common.
  - o <u>Why it happens:</u> While pregnancy and

childbirth are the source of damage to the pelvic floor, decreasing estradiol levels and increasing weight are to blame for increasing urinary incontinence. The lining of the urethra and base of the bladder are very sensitive to the effects of estradiol. Like the vagina, low estradiol levels mean that blood flow is reduced to the tissue and the tissue thins. Low estradiol levels can also contribute to reduced muscle tone in the pelvic floor, which can lead to increased urinary leakage. Abdominal fat increases pressure inside the abdomen and on the bladder, thus leading to increased urinary leakage. The percentage of menopausal females that have episodes of urinary incontinence is 30-40%

- <u>Options:</u>
  - Reduce weight by 5-10% in those with BMI above 25
  - Increase pelvic muscle supporting exercise: squats and lunges
  - Pelvic floor physical therapy
  - Stop smoking
  - Improve sleep
  - Increase walking
  - Tai chi, Yoga
  - Acupuncture or acupressure
  - Avoid nightshades, citrus, coffee, alcohol,

and artificial sweeteners

- Prescription therapy (off-label usage): estrogens, onabotulinum toxin, imipramine, or duloxetine
- Prescription therapy (approved): antimuscarinics (like Ditropan, Detrol, or Enablex) or Mirabegron

- Hair growth in unwanted places
  - <u>The Scenario:</u> I'm sure you are familiar with the "older lady" in your family or at church with long hairs on her chin and neck. Nothing is more horrifying than discovering the first one on your chin or neck! Increasing thick terminal hairs and the return of acne are not unusual during menopause. A general rule of thumb is that women who had these issues as young women are likely to have them again during and after the transition to menopause. If you had very little worrisome hair growth on your face or very little acne during your teen years, you are much less likely to have those become an issue during menopause.

  - <u>Why it happens:</u> Increasing terminal hair growth and acne are signs of testosterone influence. Before menopause, high levels of circulating estradiol generally blocked or suppressed the effects of your natural testosterone levels and even more importantly, high levels of sex hormone binding globulin (SHBG), stored testosterone, and other hormones in an inactive state in the blood. With reduced estradiol, there is less SHBG and more free testosterone available to act upon hair follicles and skin cells.

- Options:
  - Reduce testosterone supplementation
  - Weight loss
  - Prescription therapy (approved): eflornithine, spironolactone
  - Laser hair removal
  - Waxing
  - Shaving
  - Tweezing
  - Epilation
  - Depilatory creams
  - Threading
  - Electrolysis
  - Herbal or nutraceutical: spearmint, turmeric, chasteberry, tea tree oil, saw palmetto, black cohosh

- Hair loss in unwanted places
  - <u>Description</u>: Your hairdresser may be the first to notice increased hair loss and shedding and areas of thinning at the top of your head. Similar to postpartum occurrences, significant shifts in hormonal balance can have a profound effect on the hair follicles.

  - <u>Why it happens:</u> Typically, a sustained combined drop in estrogens and progesterone can trigger hair follicles to synchronize into a shedding phase. Because scalp hair takes so long to grow, significant hair loss is noticeable. During the transition to menopause, hormone levels do not rebound like they did postpartum. Low estradiol leads to the decrease of blood flow to the hair follicles. Inflammation around the hair follicles can increase, and the hair follicles can be inhibited from returning to a growth phase. This can lead to permanent thinning of the scalp hair.

  - <u>Options:</u>
    - Regular sleep schedule
    - Regular eating schedule
    - Stress reduction
    - Maintain good hydration
    - Achieve normal ferritin (iron) levels

- Increase protein intake in diet
- Increase olive/olive oil intake
- Reduce testosterone supplementation
- Prescription therapy (approved): minoxidil, finasteride, or spironolactone
- Scalp massage
- Stop chemical hair treatments (dye, bleach, and perms)
- Stop hair styling that requires traction: wigs, extensions, braids, or ponytails
- Aromatherapy: rosemary, peppermint, thyme, or cedarwood
- Herbal or nutraceutical: biotin, hyaluronic acid, flax seeds, rosemary, or chia seeds

- **Constipation**
  - <u>Description:</u> You may not realize it, but constipation can be a common occurrence during the transition to menopause. It sounds counterintuitive because higher levels of progesterone are associated with constipation. The movement of your intestines is dependent upon the proper transmission of signals in the neural (nerve) network of the intestinal tract.

  - <u>Why it happens:</u> Just like in the brain, this neural network is highly sensitive to the effects of estradiol.

Decreased estradiol can limit functioning of the intestinal neural network and shift the normal balance of bacteria that live in the gut. These factors along with decreasing hydration, sleep interruption, and decreased physical activity combine to slow intestinal motility and cause constipation.

- Options:
  - Regular sleep schedule
  - Regular eating schedule
  - Stress reduction
  - Maintain good hydration
  - Optimize whole foods in diet
  - Increased uncooked versions of whole foods in your diet
  - Decrease processed food in your diet
  - Increase fiber intake
  - Increase physical activity
  - Over-the-counter: laxatives or stool softeners
  - Prescription therapy (approved): prucalopride, lactitol, naloxegol, naldemedine
  - Abdominal massage
  - Enema
  - Aromatherapy: lemon, peppermint, ginger, or marjoram

- Herbal or nutraceutical: psyllium husk, fennel, lemon, marjoram, peppermint, ginger, vanilla, chia seed, or inulin

QUESTIONS

<u>Can you test my hormones to see what stage of menopause I am in?</u>

Hormonal testing is not as helpful in determining one's stage in menopause as you may think. When most women get hormone testing to assess menopause, they are generally getting their levels of FSH and LH tested. As discussed before, these are the chemical signals your brain sends out to control how much estradiol the ovaries produce and to stimulate ovulation. These levels naturally change every few days during the normal menstrual cycle. During the menopause transition, FSH and LH levels can fluctuate significantly from month to month.

Factors to consider in women 40 and over:
- When FSH levels are below 15, regardless of LH levels, this is indicative of ongoing ovulation. For a woman in the normal age range who has skipped multiple cycles and has menopausal symptoms, this does not mean that she hasn't entered the early stages of her transition to menopause. It does mean that there is a likelihood of pregnancy, and the situation needs monitoring.
- When FSH and LH levels are near zero, this indicates a problem with the signaling from the brain and is not likely to

be associated with menopause.
- When FSH and LH levels are simultaneously higher than 40, it indicates that menopause has been achieved.
- Testing for hormone levels is simply not a reliable tool for determining your stage in menopause.

Are there any medications or treatments for menopause?

No, menopause is a natural process and not a disease to be treated. Symptoms of menopause that are bothersome or debilitative in your life can be addressed through various methods. Depending on the symptom or complaint in question, you can use herbal formulas, alternative medicine therapies, hormonal therapy, other prescription therapies, or other non-medicinal therapeutic techniques for relief. Existing disease processes can worsen during the transition to menopause and therefore may need to be treated or you may need to have existing treatments adjusted.

What are the long-term health risks of menopause?

Menopause is a natural process in a woman's life. The shift to a low hormone environment is accompanied by profound changes in your body. One of the motivations for medical science to "do something" about menopause is to address the changes that interfere with women functioning at their healthiest level throughout their lives.

The most concerning long-term changes in regard to menopause are:

1) The increase in cardiovascular disease risks
- Atherosclerotic vascular disease that leads to stroke and heart attacks
- Heart failure, mainly associated with poorly treated high blood pressure
- Heart disease associated with arrhythmias and heart valve disease

2) The increase in bone loss

3) The cognitive changes that increase dementia risks

4) The increase in inflammatory conditions

5) The changes to metabolism and insulin resistance that lead to increased diabetes and ongoing weight gain

6) The changes to muscle tone that impact mobility and physical activity

7) The changes to pelvic function and support that impair urinary and fecal continence

8) The changes to vulvar and vaginal tissues that lead to impaired sexual function

Can I still have children after menopause?

Achieving menopause implies that there are no longer any eggs available to develop and be fertilized for pregnancy. If you are wanting to still have children, then consultation with specialists in assisted reproduction is best. Achieving menopause by completing 12 continuous months without a menstrual cycle makes it unlikely that you will ovulate again. If you are not wanting future pregnancy, continuing contraceptive practices until you are fully postmenopausal (that is two years after your last cycle) is the safest practice. Almost 10% of women will have another menstrual cycle in the 12-18 months after their "last menstrual cycle". Persistent bleeding, repetitive bleeding, or non-menstrual bleeding that occurs after you have gone a year without a cycle should be evaluated by your gynecologist.

Why don't they prepare us for menopause?

Teaching menopause is not the same as going to the public school "sex education" classes we all had in 7th and 8th grades. There is no learning institution in which all adults participate, so it would be impossible to provide learning for menopause in the same manner in which we learned about puberty. The lack of preparation for menopause falls into three main categories:

1) Most of us are not living a multigenerational family existence anymore. We no longer live our daily adult lives around the women in the family who are older and have completed menopause. What's missing is witnessing the lived experience of menopause as a normal part of life.

2) Another aspect of the sense of being unprepared

is the reality that learning about menopause is not a priority before one gets closer to the normal age range of menopause. Women in their 20s and 30s are primarily concerned with getting pregnant or making sure they don't get pregnant. Teenagers are certainly not interested in or prepared to talk about menopause.

3) Publicly speaking about "female issues" has been a taboo in most communities. Many women feel a degree of shame and a need for secrecy associated with their menstrual cycles.

The notion of freely discussing menopause is gaining momentum. The internet and social media make it so much easier for women to access information. I want this book to be part of that database of information.

How do I know when I start my menopause transition?

You will not know the exact day that you start the menopause transition, but two factors indicate that you are in the midst of it: symptoms and changes in your menstrual cycle. The most common and recognized symptom is hot flashes/vasomotor symptoms. Vaginal discomfort due to decreased lubrication and "mood" changes like increased irritability and worsening PMS are other common symptoms. The changes in your menstrual cycle include skipped cycles, a more than 7 day change in how often your cycles occur, and a reduction in the amount of flow during your cycle.

<u>Can I take something to help my menopausal symptoms even though my cycles are regular, and my hormone levels are "normal"?</u>

Yes, you can. There are quite a few options with regard to herbal and nutraceutical preparations that may provide significant relief from menopausal symptoms in the early stages. You can also start hormone replacement therapy for more severe symptoms. It is important that you understand that the doses of hormone needed to help with menopausal symptoms is much lower than that needed to protect against pregnancy. Do not assume that being on hormones means you can't get pregnant during this phase of your menopause transition.

<u>Why does my physician get upset when they find out I get hormones or take herbs provided by someone else?</u>

An upset physician is generally an uncomfortable physician. There are two aspects to this. Your physician is medically and legally liable for the care they provide. When you have a care plan from someone else, they are responsible for fully caring for you. The proliferation of anti-aging spas and centers lends itself to a level of inadequately monitored care being available in many communities. Getting your hormones or herbal preparations from another provider and then asking your physician to order labs or tests to support what the other provider is doing is not appropriate. Your physician is responsible for addressing the results of any test they order. Your physician may be afraid to refuse your request, but they certainly resent being put in a position of liability to support the care you are paying someone else to provide.

    The other aspect of being uncomfortable is that your physician may not agree with the care plan or have concerns with the long-term safety of your care plan. Quite often, women will initiate care with someone that requires full cash payment and when financial limitations occur, go to their physician to request that they refill medications and continue the care plan. Your physician is not responsible for maintaining a treatment plan with which they don't agree or that they don't provide. That is worthy of a discussion with your physician to make sure you and her/him are on the same page. Getting a full understanding of what your physician is able and willing to provide in support of your menopause transition is very important.

<u>How will I know I'm in menopause if I'm on birth control pills or hormonal contraception?</u>

    You may not know. There are many women on birth control pills/oral contraceptives still having regular cycles and not showing any signs of menopause. Between ages 40 and 50, it is wise to have a discussion with your physician about the risks and benefits of remaining on your current oral contraceptive formula. For women on long-acting hormonal contraception like Mirena, Kyleena, Skyla, Liletta, or Nexplanon, menstrual cycles may not occur. Around age 50, if you have no signs or symptoms of menopause, it is important to have a discussion with your physician about how and when to check your hormone levels to monitor for the completion of menopause. It is perfectly reasonable to discuss sterilization for you (or your husband/significant other) in order to stop hormonal contraception before there is proof of menopause.

How will I know I'm in menopause if I've had a hysterectomy or endometrial ablation?

Menopausal symptoms are the best indication of the menopause transition in women who have had their uterus removed or the lining of the uterus ablated. If there are no menopausal symptoms by age 50, have a discussion with your physician regarding if or when to check your hormone levels to monitor for the completion of menopause. Remember, menopause is a natural transformation. If you are having no symptoms or problems and you have no ability to get pregnant, then there is no medical need to monitor the exact occurrence of menopause.

When is the safest time to start hormones?

Menopausal hormone therapy can begin as soon as bothersome symptoms occur. It can begin even though you are still having some menstrual cycles but should be started no later than 10 years after the final menstrual cycle. Women under 60 years old have the least negative risk from usage.

If I have high blood pressure, can I take hormones?

Estrogens and testosterones are known to increase blood pressure. High blood pressure (hypertension) is considered a relative contraindication to estrogen therapy. That means there is a risk that taking the hormones may worsen your hypertension. If hypertension is uncontrolled, taking hormone therapy may cause more harm to you than the relief it may provide from menopausal symptoms.

Are all herbs safe to take?

No. Just because something is herbal or natural, doesn't make it safe to use. It is important to be aware that there are some herbs that can cause liver damage. There are many herbs that can interfere with the safe dosing levels of other medications like blood thinners or blood pressure medications. Some herbal preparations may have toxic contaminants or heavy metals. Excessive doses of vitamin or herbal preparations can also be harmful. Just as with medications, the risks and benefits of using a particular herbal preparation should always be assessed. Obtaining quality herbal preparations from sources that can provide consistent and uncontaminated dosing is essential.

Can menopause cause pain?

Pain is a very general symptom. Increased migraine headaches can occur in many women during the menopause transition. (Interestingly, many women experience relief from migraine headaches once they complete their menopause transition.) There are certainly many times I had patients complain of "aching bones" during their menopausal transition. We know that there is a significant loss of bone in the first five years after the final menstrual cycle. Reports of joint aches have also been noted. There are subtle changes in the immune system that may account for this complaint. Having increased cramps, back pain, abdominal pain, etc, is not typically associated with the menstrual transition.

Can menopause affect my breast health? How can I maintain my breast health during menopause?

Yes. Hormonally responsive tissue, like breast tissue, can become noticeably smaller and less plump as low hormone levels persist. These changes do NOT increase the likelihood of breast cancer. Most breast cancer risk factors are associated with obesity, specific types of hormone usage, excessive alcohol usage, radiation exposure, pregnancy history, family history, and breast-feeding history. Continue routine self breast exams often enough to be familiar with what your breasts normally feel like, continue routine mammograms every other year until at least age 74.

<u>Can menopause lead to changes in body odor?</u>

Yes. Body odor is a complex occurrence of factors that include the interplay of hormones in stimulating sweat and sebum glands to secrete. These secretions are then acted upon by normal skin bacteria to produce aromas. Decreased hormone levels can alter the secretion of these glands leading to changes in skin bacteria and "odors."

<u>What can my husband/significant other do to help me through menopause?</u>

My best advice has always been for them to understand that it is not about them, it's about YOU. YOU are undergoing a massive and radical transformation to your whole being. It is not something to be fixed. They need to be understanding. They need to be patient. Most importantly, they need to lighten your load. Clean the house, do the cooking, handle the kids, do the laundry, wear winter pajamas and stop complaining about being cold, stop acting like the change in sexual pattern means you don't love them and are having an affair…I could go on. Your menopause transition is very unsettling to the people closest to you, especially your partner. This is a time during which you question everything about your personal life and health and future. This is not a time to attack and belittle and get revenge for all prior hurts. This is not a time to make radical and final life decisions.

THE EMOTIONAL PART

MENOPAUSE IS SCARY!! It's one thing to understand the process of this transition, but most women worry about how they will experience these changes. If you are terrified about menopause, you are not alone. So much of the information that is available about menopause is limited to the physical changes. The truly scary part of menopause is the emotional and psychological side. What does achieving menopause mean to you? How do you feel about the end of your fertility? How do you feel about getting older? How do you feel about yourself at this stage in your life?

Menopause may make you think that everything happening to you at this stage in your life is hormonal, but it also occurs at the same time as midlife for women. Other aspects of your body are declining naturally due to advancing years; some due to poor health. Your life responsibilities and realities are also a factor at this time. You are in your peak earning years financially. You have accumulated 25-35 years of adulthood experiences that play a role in your current home life, social life, and work life. You are living the results of decision-making over these past few decades and understanding that the decisions you make now, will have a profound impact on these next, final 25-35 years of your life.

- Menopause does **NOT** mean you are **OLD** or **FINISHED**.

    I looked up the definition of "old" and saw words like ancient, worn-out, discarded, broken down, and tiresome. How depressing! We live in a society that prizes youth with its strength and inexperience over age with its perseverance and wisdom. It can be very difficult to embrace the natural changes in life that happen in middle age, because you fear being discarded, being considered ancient, and being thought of as old. Understanding and adjusting your outlook on what it means to achieve menopause and middle age is crucial to your success in this transition. So much of the association of being old, worn out or ancient during menopause happened because life expectancy after menopause used to be only about 10-15 years. In our modern society, life expectancy after menopause is very likely an additional 30-45 years. That is almost the same amount of time you spent between puberty and menopause. That's a game-changing number of years to exist beyond fertility. What you do with that time is crucial. Will you just exist? Will you just passively fade away, or will you make it your business to live the life you intended to live all along? When I looked up the definition of "old", I also saw phrases like long-standing, persisting from an earlier time, experienced, familiar over time, and vintage. How will you embrace menopause?

- Menopause does **NOT** mean you are **UNDESIRABLE** or **DISPENSABLE.**

    Menopause means you are no longer fertile. It does not mean that you no longer have a place in life. So many women believe that the only reason for their existence is to produce babies or provide sexual pleasure. Your existence on the earth is not limited to what goes into or comes out of your vagina. The challenge for you is to dispel the messages that society sends out about the value of women. Women are the ONLY creatures who can produce more humans. Understanding that fact is empowering. Menopause allows you to influence how this entire world functions without also being in the midst of human reproduction. It is important that you wake up to that reality. Embrace the opportunity to impact life on a whole new level.

- Menopause does **NOT** mean you are **BROKEN** or **CRAZY**.

    You may feel like you are going crazy, but you aren't. It is very unsettling to feel such a lack of control over what is happening to you and your behavior during this transition to menopause. The feeling of not being in control of who you typically are is very discouraging.

Struggling to focus and complete tasks that didn't previously even require you to think is scary. Feeling absolutely overwhelmed with the changes and the fear of these changes is enough to send you over the edge. Do not struggle, worry or despair. Get help if you are overwhelmed. Get treatment if you are unable to function adequately in your life. It is perfectly normal for you to be unhappy with how you are feeling. These changes are not a figment of your imagination. YOU ARE NOT CRAZY!

- Menopause does mean that **FERTILITY HAS ENDED**.

  Whether you are relieved, devastated, or indifferent, menopause means the end of natural spontaneous fertility. There'll be no more babies, because you have run out of eggs. There is such a finality about that and it can be very emotionally intense. For women who haven't had control of their fertility, it is a welcome relief and a godsend. For women who have struggled and been unsuccessful in conceiving, it is the deepest of spiritual blows. Many women find themselves mourning the loss of fertility without any desire to actually have additional children. Respect the change and acknowledge your feelings. Know that you are not alone.

- Menopause does mean that **YOUR BODY HAS CHANGED**.

    No more cycles, no more menstrual cramping, and no more PMS. No more pads, tampons, and menstrual cups. You may experience dryness everywhere, along with personal summers and personal rages. You name it, things have changed. These changes come with the territory. Just like puberty, you've crossed into a new world. Your ability to embrace this change and use it to propel you to a healthier and more satisfying life is the challenge.

- Menopause does mean that **YOU ARE STILL ALIVE**.

    You have survived and made it to this age and this time in your life. It is a time of rejoicing. Do not allow yourself to fall victim to the societal negatives about women and aging. This is the opportunity of a lifetime. While it is not a do-over, it is a reset. How you choose to approach this transition will make all the difference in the world.

Conclusion

You may be thinking that I just shared the names of some treatments, but I didn't tell you how to use them. Well, there are two reasons for that:

1) Menopause is a natural process in a woman's life. It does not get treated. Symptoms may be bothersome, and it is your decision to address that, or not. If symptoms are mild, typically you can try things available to you at home or over the counter. This book gives you information about the multitude of things you can do for yourself. I do not give dosing or formulation options because there are simply too many available to list here. If symptoms are significant, seeing your physician or healthcare provider for help that can include prescription options is best. Risk factors for or the presence of medical conditions need to be taken into account when addressing more significant symptoms. Weight loss, changes in lifestyle, intentional nutrition, and increased physical activity are the cornerstones of maintaining health after changes occur to your body during menopause.

2) Outlining specific treatments for a specific problem is considered part of the practice of medicine. This is an educational guide about menopause and it does not provide any diagnoses or treatments. In order to get the optimal treatment

for significant symptoms, your individual needs, concerns, and risk factors need to be assessed. Once a treatment plan has been set up, there needs to be a follow-up to ensure that it is successful. You should be monitored to make sure there are no side effects or health risks with continuing treatment. There needs to be a mechanism to safely change the treatment plan, or stop it, as time goes on.

Let me give you SEVEN reasons to embrace menopause:

1) No more menstrual cycles, tampons, anemia, cramps, or PMS.

2) No more pregnancies or fear of pregnancy. No more contraception!

3) Granny mode vs. GLAMMA mode! You get to decide. You are not at the end of your life and stuck at home watching grandkids.

4) You can now freely do all the things you snuck around trying to do as a teen without getting into trouble. You've got your own place, car, and money, and can do what you want to do!

5) There's plenty of time left to live the life you intended to live.

6) You and your partner are empty nesters and can get back to being boyfriend and girlfriend, again.

7) Your career is in full swing and can wind down or keep trucking along!

Reference Lists

Hormones

Types of hormonal preparations

- Oral (tablet)
- Topical/Transdermal (cream, patch, or gel)
- Sublingual (rapidly dissolving mini-pellet or troche)
- Injection
- Intravaginal (cream, gel, or suppository)
- Subcutaneous (pellet)
- Intrauterine device

Side effect profile for estrogens

- Risk of stroke
- Risk of pulmonary embolism
- Risk of breast cancer
- Risk of endometrial cancer
- Risk of increased fibroid growth
- Risk of weight gain
- Risk of hypertension

- Risk of kidney failure
- Risk of polycythemia

Specific Hormones

- Estradiol
- Estrone
- Estriol
- Conjugated estrogens
- Progesterone
- Progestins
- Pregnenolone
- DHEA
- Testosterone

Herbal Options

- Red clover
- Red raspberry leaf
- Rhubarb
- Evening primrose
- Soy isoflavones
- Ginseng
- Gingko
- Dong quai
- Black cohosh
- Flaxseed oil
- Borage oil
- Chasteberry (Vitex)
- Horny goat weed
- Fenugreek
- Tribulus
- MACA
- Lion's Mane
- Rosemary
- Psyllium
- Licorice
- Valerian root
- Chamomile
- Lemon balm
- Lavender

- Fennel
- Spearmint

Dietary supplements

- Vitamin C
- Vitamin D3
- Vitamin B1 (thiamine)
- Vitamin B2 (riboflavin)
- Vitamin B3 (niacin)
- Vitamin B5 (pantothenic acid)
- Vitamin B6 (pyridoxine)
- Vitamin B7 (biotin)
- Vitamin B9 (folate)
- Vitamin B12 (cobalamin)
- Vitamin K2
- Vitamin A
- Turmeric
- Omega III
- Co-enzyme Q10

Nutraceutical Options

- Antioxidants
- Resveratrol
- Green tea
- ECGC (green tea extract)
- DIM
- Ashwagandha
- Rhodiola
- Curcumin (turmeric)
- Co-Enzyme Q10
- L-Theanine
- 5-Hydroxytryptophan
- MACA
- Lion's Mane
- Reishi Mushroom
- Soy isoflavones
- Melatonin
- Cannabinol (CBN)
- Cannabidiol (CBD)

Non-Pharmaceutical Remedies

- Yoga
- Tai chi
- Pilates
- Exercise
- Weight training
- Walking
- Acupuncture
- Cranial electrical stimulation
- Sleep devices
- Laser vaginal rejuvenation
- Plasma-rich platelet subcutaneous injections
- Stellate ganglion block for hot flashes
- Acupressure devices
- Pelvic floor physical therapy
- Sleep apnea correction
- Cooling devices

RESOURCES

9 Tips for a Successful Physician Visit

1. Be clear about what you need. Your physician is not a mind reader. Tell her/him if you need:
    a. help with symptoms
    b. information about menopause
    c. reassurance that what's happening with you is normal
    d. any or all of the above
2. Know your personal medical history.
    a. Write down the details.
    b. Write down all medicines and supplements you use.
    c. Take the list with you to the visit.
3. Write your questions down and bring them with you to the visit. Don't forget to ask any questions you may have about your period or about risk of pregnancy.
4. Make a Symptom list. List the symptoms in order of how badly they disrupt your life. Take the list with you to the visit. Use that same original list to document improvement (or not) in symptoms over time.
5. Know your family medical history. Write down the details.

Include your parents, siblings, children, grandparents, aunts and uncles.
6. Call ahead to find out if your physician is comfortable managing menopause. Can you get scheduled for a full 30 or 45 or 60 minute talk visit? Is s/he flexible and knowledgeable regarding treatment options?
7. Track your menstrual cycles and bleeding days in a journal, calendar or menstrual tracking app. Bring that information with you to each visit.
8. Think about the types of treatment that you prefer. Would you like hormones, do you hate the thought of anything herbal, do you have sensitive skin and can't tolerate patches or topical creams? All of those things count.
9. Be clear about what you prefer in terms of treatment but remain open to other options in case what you want is not safe for you or doesn't work for you.

Cycle Calendar

Mark each day of your cycle. Make a note about anything unusual about the cycle. Make note of any menopausal symptoms you notice. Take your calendar with you to each visit.

Menstrual Cycle Calendar

JANUARY 2024

SUN	MON	TUE	WED	THU	FRI	SAT
	1	2	3	4	5	6
7	8	9	10	11	12	13
14	15	16	17	18	19	20
21	22	23	24	25	26	27
28	29	30	31			

FEBRUARY 2024

SUN	MON	TUE	WED	THU	FRI	SAT
				1	2	3
4	5	6	7	8	9	10
11	12	13	14	15	16	17
18	19	20	21	22	23	24
25	26	27	28	29		

MARCH 2024

SUN	MON	TUE	WED	THU	FRI	SAT
					1	2
3	4	5	6	7	8	9
10	11	12	13	14	15	16
17	18	19	20	21	22	23
24	25	26	27	28	29	30
31						

Notes

APRIL 2024

SUN	MON	TUE	WED	THU	FRI	SAT
	1	2	3	4	5	6
7	8	9	10	11	12	13
14	15	16	17	18	19	20
21	22	23	24	25	26	27
28	29	30				

MAY 2024

SUN	MON	TUE	WED	THU	FRI	SAT
			1	2	3	4
5	6	7	8	9	10	11
12	13	14	15	16	17	18
19	20	21	22	23	24	25
26	27	28	29	30	31	

JUNE 2024

SUN	MON	TUE	WED	THU	FRI	SAT
						1
2	3	4	5	6	7	8
9	10	11	12	13	14	15
16	17	18	19	20	21	22
23	24	25	26	27	28	29
30						

Notes

_____
_____
_____
_____

JULY 2024

SUN	MON	TUE	WED	THU	FRI	SAT
	1	2	3	4	5	6
7	8	9	10	11	12	13
14	15	16	17	18	19	20
21	22	23	24	25	26	27
28	29	30	31			

AUGUST 2024

SUN	MON	TUE	WED	THU	FRI	SAT
				1	2	3
4	5	6	7	8	9	10
11	12	13	14	15	16	17
18	19	20	21	22	23	24
25	26	27	28	29	30	31

SEPTEMBER 2024

SUN	MON	TUE	WED	THU	FRI	SAT
1	2	3	4	5	6	7
8	9	10	11	12	13	14
15	16	17	18	19	20	21
22	23	24	25	26	27	28
29	30					

Notes

OCTOBER 2024

SUN	MON	TUE	WED	THU	FRI	SAT
		1	2	3	4	5
6	7	8	9	10	11	12
13	14	15	16	17	18	19
20	21	22	23	24	25	26
27	28	29	30	31		

NOVEMBER 2024

SUN	MON	TUE	WED	THU	FRI	SAT
					1	2
3	4	5	6	7	8	9
10	11	12	13	14	15	16
17	18	19	20	21	22	23
24	25	26	27	28	29	30

DECEMBER 2024

SUN	MON	TUE	WED	THU	FRI	SAT
1	2	3	4	5	6	7
8	9	10	11	12	13	14
15	16	17	18	19	20	21
22	23	24	25	26	27	28
29	30	31				

Notes

Menopause Symptom Tracker

Make a list of the worrisome symptoms you are experiencing. Write them down in order from the most bothersome symptom to the least bothersome one. If you could only get one symptom relieved, which one would it be? That should be the first symptom you write down. If that first symptom is relieved, what would be the next symptom that I must have fixed? That would be the second symptom you write down.

Next to each symptom, assign a number to indicate how badly the symptom is bothering you or disrupting your life: 1 for mild, 2 for moderate, 3 for significant, 4 for severe.

Take your symptom list with you to each visit. Once you have started some type of intervention to relieve your symptom, refer to your symptom list to see what has changed, improved, or gone away. Write this down on your original list and keep following to remind yourself of your progress.

Menopause Symptoms

Description	Severity

About the Author

Donna G Ivery, MD has done all things women's health, delivering babies, rocking surgeries, and championing the cause for almost 30 years. Beginning with training in Atlanta, to the tropical islands of Maui, Hawaii, and St. Croix, to the lively streets of Portland, small towns in Georgia, and her homebase of Titusville, Florida, Dr Donna G MD has been a guiding light for over 50,000 women throughout her illustrious career.

Dr Donna G MD started professional life as a biomedical engineering graduate of Johns Hopkins University and an employee of AT&T Bell Labs. She pivoted to medicine with medical school and residency training in Obstetrics & Gynecology at Emory in Atlanta, GA, marking the beginning of a remarkable career. Board-certified in Obstetrics & Gynecology since 1998 and certified in Integrative Holistic Medicine since 2014, she has seamlessly blended conventional and holistic approaches to provide comprehensive care to her patients.

Beyond the accolades of a thriving clinical practice, Dr. Donna G MD shares a deeply personal narrative. She has been through the wringer at times in her life, too — exhausted, sick, overweight and feeling completely overwhelmed. Sound familiar? Yeah, Dr Donna G MD knows what it's like to hit the wall, be forced to change course, and figure out how to move forward. She was diagnosed with Multiple

Sclerosis over 25 years ago and it reared its ugly head in 2019!! While struggling to recover, the COVID pandemic hit and life became a blur and a blessing. You see, Dr Donna G MD knows life without maternity leave and went back to work 3 ½ weeks after her c-section. COVID's silver lining gave her the bonding with her son that she missed postpartum! Great physicians and nurses along with great modern medicines all contributed to getting a grateful Dr Donna G MD back on her feet and functioning.

So, here's the scoop: Dr Donna G MD's mission in 2024 is to reach a million amazing women with the Message About Menopause. This book is a big part of reaching that goal!

Why do something like this? Because so many women are completely unprepared for menopause. They don't know what to expect. They are afraid of what is happening to their body and their mind. They are confused about all of the information and mixed messages they see on the internet. Dr Donna G MD spent decades helping women, one by one, through their gynecologic issues, especially menopause. Some got information, some got hormones, some got herbal regimens, some got practical and nutritional advice and tips; they all got seen and heard and helped in a manner that resonated with their experience and needs. With five decades of life experience, she intimately understands the challenges women face – the struggle to be heard, believed, and helped.

Website: Https://www.drdonnagmd.com

Podcast: https://drdonnagmd.exposure.co

Email: DrDonnaGMD@femalematters.com

Youtube: @DrDonnaGMD655

Tiktok: @DrDonnaGMD

Facebook/Instagram: @DrDonnaGMD

LinkedIN: @DrDonnaGMD

Join the Movement

#messageaboutmenopause

#notyourgrannysmenopause

1. Post a picture on social media of you with the book and tag me @DrDonnaGMD
2. Buy someone else a copy of the book and give it as a gift.
3. Feature the book in your book club.
4. Ask your local bookstore to carry the book.
5. Book me to speak at your next event - www.drdonnagmd.com"

Made in the USA
Columbia, SC
09 June 2024